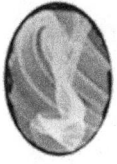

Energy Healing 101

A Primer for Novices with Tips for the Advanced

Connie Dohan

Energy Healing 101

(A Primer for Novices with Tips for the Advanced)

The author may be contacted through

Connie@AmidAngels.com

Connie is an energy intuitive and seer. She is a gifted healer as well as a talented teacher and speaker.

She was not born this way, but rather grew into it. Her training was initially the school of life where infirmity and unanswered questions forced her to look for solutions "outside the box". Because of this, her writing and teaching is understandable and easily applicable by all — especially the beginner and the one at "a fork" in one's life's path.

She has a practice in Ohio where she specializes in metaphysical weight loss, energy healing, soul's calling counseling, private teaching, and mentoring. She is available for speaking or lecturing on a variety of topics.

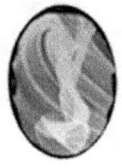

Energy Healing 101

A Primer for Novices with Tips for the Advanced

Connie Dohan

Dedicated to Bill –
my husband, my lover, my best friend,
my soul mate, my confidant,
my holder of light at the end of every dark tunnel

Table of Contents

Energy Healing 101

A Primer for the Novice with Tips for the Advanced

Introduction

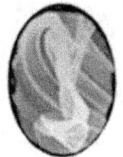

So, you have taken your first energy healing class — Reiki, Quantum Touch, EFT, Chios or any of a myriad of the others out there.

Or maybe you have graduated from a class but have been only practicing on your cat, dog, parrot or other unsuspecting pet. Or, maybe you are practicing on quietly on close friends or family. How do you take it from family, pets, and friends to "real" clients?

Perhaps you have been practicing energy healing for some time now but are not getting paid enough (or at all) for the sessions you do.

How do those other people do it? What are the "tips of the trade" that make certain people in the trade stand out as a notch above?

What takes a healer from an amateur to a top notch, sought after, well paid healer?

There are unwritten tips that you can use to set yourself apart and become a confident professional in whatever modality – or combination of modalities – you choose to practice.

The writing is crisp, down to earth. It has the information you need in readily accessible form. You don't need to wade through long paragraphs to get to the one sentence you are looking for.

CHAPTER ONE
It's All About You

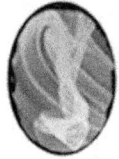

The Healer

Let us start at the beginning. Let us start with you — the healing facilitator.

Realize that no one can heal another person. Each person must be his or her own healer. You can certainly facilitate someone seeking to be healed. You can be the vessel through which healing energy flows. Only the receiver's body can be responsible for what happens to the energy once received. The receiving body processes everything on multiple levels — unconscious, subconscious and conscious. This includes healing energy. Grasping the fact that the client is the healer and you are the facilitator lets you let go of ego and lets Spirit flow.

A good example of this would be a client I saw one dreary spring day. An elderly lady, accompanied by her friend came up to see me. She complained of a sore knee and also had such a huge misshapen goiter in her throat that she had considerable trouble swallowing.

After getting her as comfortable as possible, my partner and I spent the next half hour giving her knee the very best we could. When done, we looked at her. Nothing was different about her slightly swollen knee. However, her neck area was smooth, supple and taut with a white box like marking where the goiter used to be.

Her friend was ecstatic. The client could swallow easily for the first time since the goiter had started to show. However, despite the exclamations from her friend, the client was severely put out as her knee was still sore.

You cannot predict the flow of energy or the reactions of people. It is your responsibility to give out the purest, best energy that you are capable of providing. You are not responsible for the result.

The Healer/Giver

Most energy healers are also caregivers. Most volunteer in some capacity on a regular basis.

Energy healers are just plain givers. They give 100% out and get 75% back in, often less. They just give to the point of exhaustion and then they take a breath and give some more. Giving comes naturally to a giver. They give past the point of depletion – until they are past the point of exhaustion and keep on giving.

In order to boost, rejuvenate, maintain and support a healthy being, givers and healers must support, balance, strengthen, and heal the heart chakra. This ensures giving from a place of abundance, not a place of want.

This is best done by regularly visualizing a nice emerald green on a regular basis. Just expose yourself to green as much as possible. Your body will do the rest.

Maybe you do this on a subconscious level already. Maybe your walls or wardrobe are mostly green or you surround yourself with plants. Or perhaps your signature jewelry piece is an emerald ring or a green jade bracelet. Maybe you spend a lot of time gardening or out in nature. These are all good sources of green.

Giving is a wonderful thing but most people, especially healers, need to learn to give properly. You must learn to give from a place of abundance, not a place of lack. If you are depleted, you are giving from a place of lack.

Apart from supporting your heart chakra with green, make sure you take the advice you give you give your clients. Make sure you are well rested, drink eight glasses of water a day, get enough sleep, meditate, and take time for you. Make yourself the best you that you can be. It really will affect the quality of the energy treatment you are able to give others.

Be sure to maintain your health on an energetic level as well. If you do not practice cord cutting, find it in Chapter Seven and start today. GAPS should also be part of your daily arsenal and can also be found in the same chapter.

A well rested healthy healer gives a client a much better session than does a burned out, exhausted healer.

<u>How to present</u>

Obviously, you need to dress appropriately. You cannot greet the client "looking like something the cat dragged in", as my grandfather always said. Faded blue jeans and tattered tops have no place in the healer's healing wardrobe. For females seeing males, the trinity is "no cleavage", "no cling", "no leg." Always err on the side of modesty. Wear loose, comfortable clothing or cover yourself with a lab coat.

With the number of allergies this chemical world has created, no one knows how a client might be sensitive. There is an unwritten code that practitioners not wear scents of any kind, lest the client be allergic. Scents can also trigger memories, good or bad, and potentially influence your energy session.

White

When I started, I always wore all white (or off–white) when I was healing. I still do most of the time. This serves a multitude of purposes.

1) White sets me apart as most people do not wear solid white, especially after Labor Day.
2) A person in white is most commonly thought of as being in the healing arts.
3) On some level, white always evokes a sense of honesty, cleanliness and purity.
4) White has a higher frequency than black. As such it allows energy to flow more freely, which is what you are looking for.
5) White is considered one of the angel colors, and one that you are supposed to wear when trying to attract a heavenly host. (Always helpful when doing energy work!)
6) White offers a clean palette. The client visualizing white will not have any of his or her chakras stimulated. It is like starting with a clear slate.
7) When you're trying to see auras, chakras, meridians, healing colors and angels, these are all easiest to see against a plain white backdrop.

CHAPTER TWO
Tools of the Trade

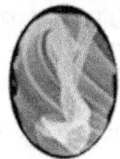

Equipment

Energy work can be done in a chair or on a table. Either way, make sure what you use is sturdy. If you are investing in a massage table, it is well worth the extra to get the equipment you know is rated for 300 pounds or more. Our population is living longer, and obesity is rising, not falling.

Avoid the worry and embarrassment of telling a client he or she is too heavy for your equipment.

If you can afford an amethyst bio–mat for your client to lie on, it is well worth the initial investment. Its infra-red rays penetrate the muscles evenly at a deep level, promoting an added level of relaxation to your treatment sessions.

Surroundings

Every attempt should be made to make the space and the things in it as neutral as possible. If color is used, be sure that all of the colors of chakra system are represented – red, orange, yellow, green, blue, violet, white.

Of course, this space should be free of distractions, noise, as well as any peculiar odors. What you consider a lovely air freshener or incense might be unpleasant or even cause headaches for others.

The space should be quiet and free from distractions – turn off the client's cell phone, as well as your own.

Lighting should be dim and subdued. Not only is this more restful for the client, this lighting is the most conducive to seeing auras and the energetic field.

Be sensitive to any music you might use; make sure it is all nature sounds or instrumental – no vocals. Words mean different things to different people.

You are trying to create a tranquil, undisturbed, safe environment for your clients.

A note about indoor fountains – while lovely to some, the sound of running water can cause the brain's natural signal for urination to kick in. So a fountain, even a small table or desk fountain, in a treatment space unknowingly can cause embarrassment as well as discomfort and should be avoided.

CHAPTER THREE
The Check "Is in the Mail"

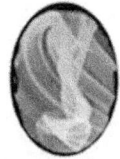

The Fee: Why, how to set it and how to collect it

The single biggest disservice novice business–minded healers/entrepreneurs do to themselves, as well as the other healers in their community or modality relates to the fee in that they do not to collect a fee, or to collect too low of a fee. Most healers are givers and giving their services is natural.

Why a Fee

The old adage is true that if you do not pay for a thing, you do not value it and its benefits will not come to pass in your life. No-one would walk into an office and walk out without paying the fee. Likewise, no-one should leave your place of healing without paying you.

Setting the Fee

Check what local practitioners in your modality are charging. At the time of writing this book, the minimum charge for area work is $1 a minute with a minimum 10 minute session.

I always charge higher – $75 an hour or more when others are at $60 an hour. I tell prospective clients up front that if they search around they will find my rates higher than anyone else but I am the best and you get what you pay for. If I was in pain, I would want the best. I have had fewer clients than my peers but more money – I am happy with that.

Collecting the Fee

For many healers, collecting the fee is the most difficult part of the whole process. It need not be.

1) You must see your healing gift as worthy and valuable – not to be squandered and used unwisely.

2) Realize there is a segment of our society that does not want to get well. They just want to complain and are seeking attention. There is a reason they are coming to you and not to the more seasoned healer. You listen and you give. If you don't collect a fee, you will get lots of clients, but no money.

3) Realize that while some clients spin you a sob story of impending financial doom, they have enough money for lunch out, designer jeans, a movie and other luxuries. If they applied themselves, even a little bit, they could squeeze out something for you. They do not respect you or your services if they do not pay for them.

If you do not know how to go about it, do what the pros do – post a rate fee sheet in your treatment space or print your rates on your business cards. Alternatively, you can get a sales receipt book and present your client with an invoice. That way it is like a rule and everyone knows what is expected.

I insist on prepayment – you can always have that posted on your signs too. Or you can say to your client as they are sorting out their coats and purses "Can I process your payment while you go ahead and make yourself comfortable?" or "Which method of payment will you be using?" or "Shall I take your payment now, so that we do not have to worry about it while you're all mellow after the treatment?"

Another way to deal with the money situation is to sell a package of sessions prepaid up front. This is often done by offering a small discount for the bundle.

Better the awkwardness of collecting the money beforehand and knowing you have it than wondering all throughout the session if you're going to receive the funds. Also broaching the subject at the start is definitely less awkward than trying to collect the funds after the service has been rendered.

CHAPTER FOUR
Considerations

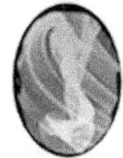

While this book addresses a general mixed practice of men and women, do not be afraid to go with your strength. If you are passionate about animals or a specific animal, by all means, set up an animal healing practice. If your forte is children or teens, specialize in that area. Even if you have a mixed general adult practice, you will most likely notice a common denominator emerging, in that most of the clients coming to you have the same problem. You will note the pattern of chronic or acute symptoms. If you look at it closer, you will notice that it is even more specifically broken down into problems of digestion, bones, eyes, etc.

Many modalities can be done either remote or live. If this is true for the one you chose, do not neglect to pursue both distant as well as local venues.

Most healers are most comfortable and most effective with modalities that they have learned and blended, or add their own flourishes, twists and touches to the broth. Do not hesitate to "mix and match" to create a system that works best for you.

Chakra #11

Chakra 11, often called the "Healer's Chakra", is the chakra of transmutation. Located in the soles of your feet (arches) and the palms of your hands, it is responsible for bringing in as well as giving out the energy of the energetic body. Make sure these points in your arches and palms are open and cleared. If not or if in doubt, simply massaging these spots yourself will be sufficient to open and clear them.

Massaging your third eye will also aid in opening it up so that you can tune in more to your clients' needs and how to meet them.

Tools

Some healing modalities work with energy. Others like Reiki and Chios use symbols. Yet another group of modalities requires the use of tools – crystal healing and tuning forks being the most obvious.

If you are a on a budget, as most people are, remember to get the best possible tool for your money as you can. A small, accurate piece will hold you in better stead than a bigger, flashier, less accurate piece. Be sure to cleanse the tools often, especially between treatments. Follow the seller's directions for care, or if ever in doubt, just place it close to a large piece of selenite. Selenite is nature's cleanser. A large piece (log) is the surest way of cleansing anything properly.

Likewise, when not in use, your tools should be properly stored. Remember that they are fine pieces that sense/calibrate energy. If you leave them loose in a drawer or in the bottom of your purse, not only is there the probability that they will get chipped, but also there is the certainty that they will be sullied with the outside energy from their place of storage.

A nice soft bag, preferably of a natural fiber such as cotton, silk, linen or leather, will protect your tools from scratches and isolate them from outside energy.

Leather

You are sabotaging yourself before you even get out of the gate if you are not aware of the impact of leather. Know that among many of the things about energy, one critical fact is that energy is blocked by leather.

Try this little exercise. Put your arms in front of you, palms facing about twelve inches apart. Sense the energy like a little ball between them. Now run the energy back and forth like a light beam between your palms. Sense it. Now put a genuine leather glove on one hand and try to run the energy from palm to palm as previously done. Notice the difference? (You must use real leather. If you don't have leather gloves, you can wrap your hand or any other body part with a leather belt and try letting the energy run through it.)

This test was fun, but the results show that the healer cannot be connected to chakras 10 or 11 if wearing leather footwear.

In addition, energy is not free—flowing through the client if he or she is wearing leather shoes, a leather belt or has a leather wallet in his / her pocket. All these should be removed before beginning treatment. Some people wear leather watchstraps, leather hair decorations or necklaces. These too should be taken off if possible to make sure that the healer's energy is not blocked.

Touch

Most energy healing uses some form of touch in whole or in part. This should be light, without pressure or slightly off body.

Life force flows in the body as a subtle circulatory system throughout. Stress causes congestion of the life force which in turn causes dis—ease(s).

CHAPTER FIVE
Giving a Session

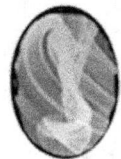

Many modalities teach you how to give the elements of the technique but not how to put it all together to be done in a session.

Once the client has paid and is comfortable, you can explain that what you are about to do is like a massage for the energy field. State that some or all of it can be done with light touch or completely off body. Give the client the option to choose hands on or hands off.

If working with the base or sacral chakra, the client may be more comfortable placing her own hand, palm down over the area and then letting you work either on or off the hand. The energy will pass through and get where it needs to be. It knows what to do.

I always tell the client that I will lightly squeeze his or her shoulder on beginning and on ending of a session. I remember going for my first massage. I became totally relaxed and oblivious to my surroundings. Then I realized I was all alone and did not know if I was done, or the masseuse had just stepped out for supplies or what was happening.

It is also helpful for the client to know that you are working with energy and will be moving energy. Belching, laughing, crying, and twitching might ensue. Reassure the client in advance that you are familiar with all this. Tell him or her to let the body clear itself, however it wants. This is a good sign.

Points to Ponder

There are a number of small but helpful tips I have picked up along the way. Each one I learned by experience as none of them were touched on in any of the books I read or classes I attended.

If your client is wearing a hearing aid and you place healing hands, even off body, near the head, the hearing aid will be activated and be sent into a high pitched squeal mode that neither you nor your client will soon forget.

If your clients are elderly or have mobility problems, getting on and off the massage table can be a challenge. A satin sheet for the massage table or even a satin runner across the center can be a big help. Satin sheets provide less friction, allowing clients more ease in movement.

When your client is lying stomach up on the massage table, go to the foot of the table, kneel down and observe the feet. Both of the feet should be parallel to each other at ninety degree angles from the floor. Most are not.

At the end of the session, look again. See how much difference your session has made (figure 1)

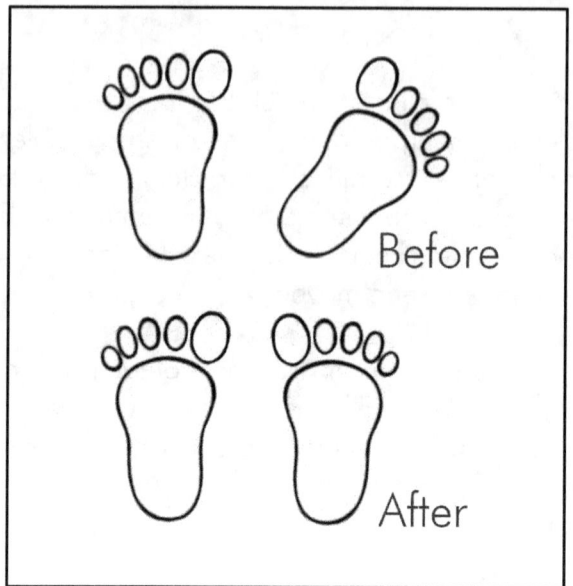

Figure 1

CHAPTER SIX
Techniques

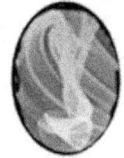

There are many different techniques from which to choose. Two of my favorites are ones I developed as a result of combining some of the healing modalities I studied. Both are good stand bys to know, easy to perform and have visible results.

I call them "Connie's Crystal Layout" and "The Green Room". I hope you will try them and use them often.

Try them out on yourself as well as your clients.

Connie's Crystal Layout

In order to do this, you will need the following:

1) Basic knowledge of some basic crystal terms listed here
2) Quartz points
3) Selenite
4) One stone for each chakra (described)

The Stones

Quartz is the Earth's most abundant mineral, and therefore inexpensive. Quartz comes in many shapes, sizes and colors. For the purposes of this layout, you will need quartz points, single terminated – the longer the better and the clearer the better (figure 2).

Selenite
1) Nature's cleanser
2) Attracts only positive energy
3) Also common and inexpensive
4) Unprocessed/raw is preferred to polished
5) Look for logs 6 inches or larger

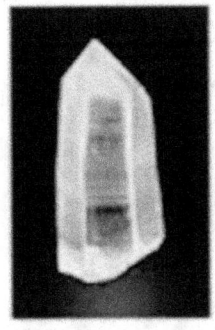

double terminated
(point on each end)

single terminated
base on one end
point on other end

Figure 2

Chakra Stones

This is where you can spend a little or spend a lot. You will need one stone for each chakra. You can read up and buy very rare or large crystals that energize each chakra. Chakra stone kits are also available. Or by knowing the colors of each chakra, you can simply get one each black, red, brown/orange, yellow, bright green, turquoise, indigo, violet, and clear stone. They need not be all smooth or even the same size.

Preparation

<u>Step 1</u>: Space Preparation
　　　Create sacred space as you normally would.

<u>Step 2</u>: Cleansing

　　　Using single terminated quartz stones, lay them out as shown in figure 3.

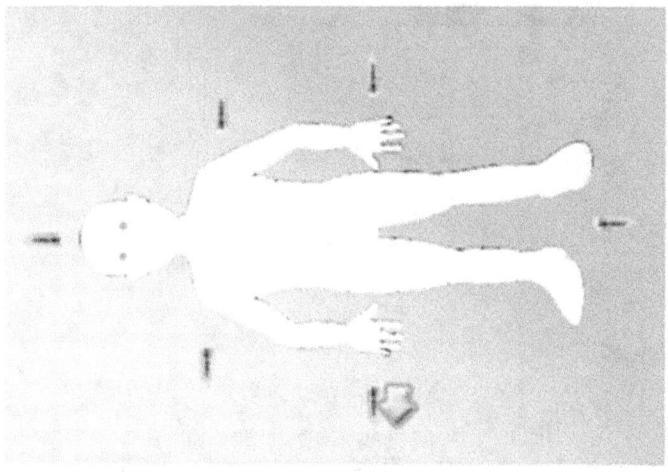

Figure 3

　　　Note each point is close to the body. The base of the point is parallel to the body. The point points away from the body. Remain this way for twenty minutes. Then remove the points.

: Fill

Place the stones on each chakra. When placing stones, do not skip about. Place them in order: 1) black, 2) red, 3) brown/orange, 4) yellow, 5) green, 6) blue, 7) indigo and 8) violet/white as in figure 4

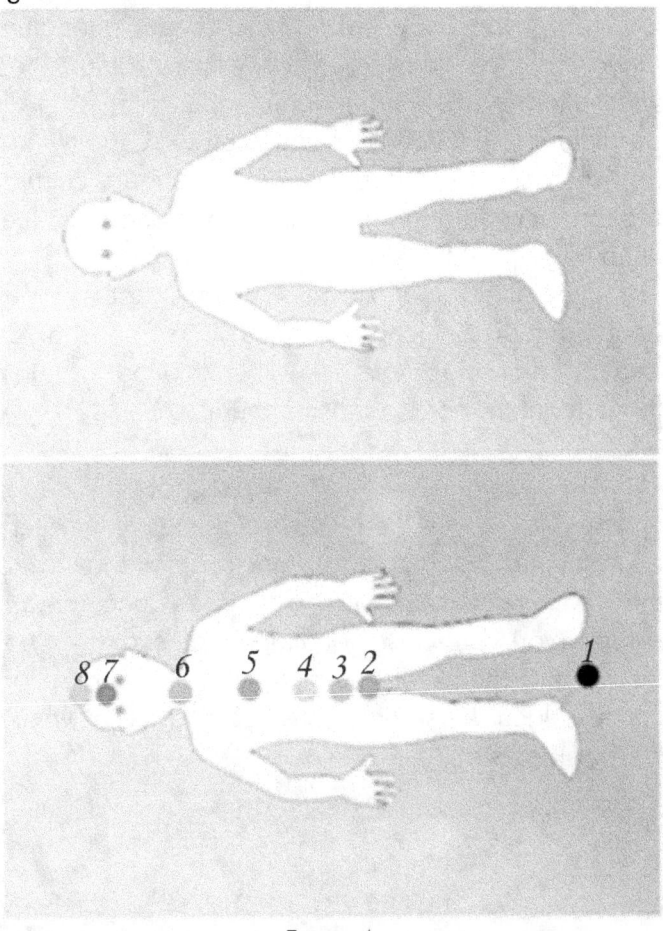

Figure 4

Note: if you do not "see" or know where each chakra is, you can easily determine this by using a pendulum. A whole book could be written on pendulums alone, but for the very basics, do the following. With client lying on table, hold your pendulum at the top of the head about six inches away from the body. Slowly move your pendulum down the face and through the entire torso. You will notice that at certain points the swing of your pendulum will change dramatically. Usually, but not always, the pendulum will spin in a circular motion. Your hand or your pendulum may feel "heavy" just before this happens.

At this point do not worry whether your pendulum gives clockwise spins for some chakras and counter clockwise for others. You are just locating them, not diagnosing them.

As well, the books always show the seven chakras in a lovely neat line. However, your client is not a book, and one or more chakras may be to the right or left of center. This is not uncommon. Again, you are just locating the chakras, not diagnosing them. If you should find a chakra off center, place the stone where you find it, not where the book says it is.

Allow the stones and the client to rest for 20 minutes. Instruct the client to rest and allow the stones just to do their thing. If they jump off or wriggle over a bit, let them do it. It is part of the process. The energy of the stone is reacting to or interacting with the energy of the client.

Advanced: If you can do all this easily, you may wish to take it one step further, or more. Try putting a double terminated quartz between each chakra stone. One point should be pointed to one chakra stone while the other is pointed to the other chakra stone.

If you can see a blockage, put the double terminated quartz only between the blocked chakras.

You will also know to place extra stones or quartz on or between certain chakras. Go ahead. What is offered here is a basic template.

After 20 minutes with the stones in place, return to your client. You may notice that the stones are in a different position. This is simply a reflection of the energy of the strong chakras interacting with the stones and will give you clues about your client's situation.

I have sessions where single stones cracked completely, took on "stains", as well as moved several inches from where they were originally placed.

Remove the stones in reverse order to the way that you placed them down - violet, indigo, green, yellow, orange/brown, red and black.

As you take each stone off, notice if any of them have heated up, cracked, or taken on a different striation or pattern. This is also a way of determining what needs to be addressed with your client.

You may want to share the changes in the stones with the client who can often comment on what possible meanings in his life might have caused the changes.

Step 4: Seal

Arrange the stones as shown in figure 5.

This time, make sure the quartz points are reversed. That is, the points are close to the body, pointing in and the base point is farthest away from the body

Place selenite logs outside the body at the base of each quartz point.

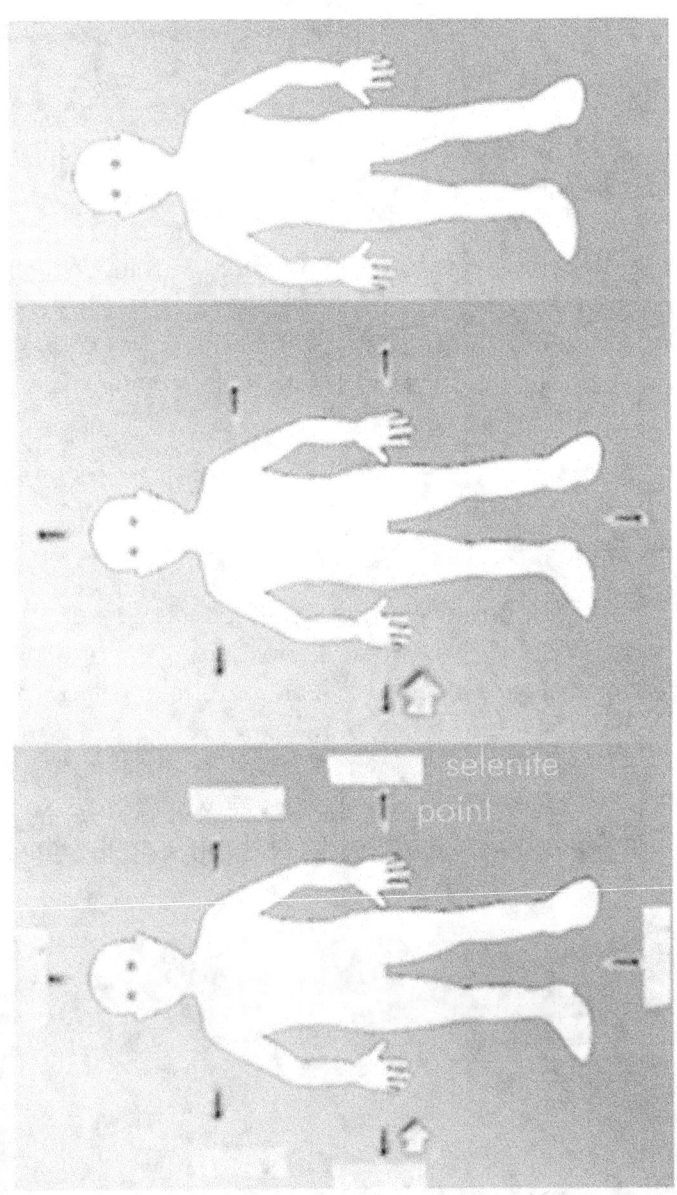

Figure 5

Allow the client to rest for 20 minutes.

You're done – the client is cleansed, filled and sealed.

This is a wonderfully rejuvenating combination of layouts. It can be easily self administered. I do it often. It is well worth carving an hour out of your schedule to experience this.

The Green Room

This powerful, hands-off technique can be done virtually anytime, anywhere. For this technique, you need a client, a regular office or kitchen chair and a box of Kleenex.

This exercise acknowledges where a person is lacking in personal power and replaces it with a sense of empowerment.

Step 1:
Let the client sit comfortably in the chair. Explain that many clients experience an emotional release at some time during the session. This is the body's way of self healing. It is normal. You, the practitioner, have seen the extremes of laughing and crying. The client should just go with flow and allow the body to express itself as it sees fit. Do not hold back.

Step 2:
Kneel in front of the client and interact with your client as follows:

"I am going to ask you to visualize a color, and while you are doing this, I am going to make some statements. If the statement is true or partially true, repeat it out loud. If the statement is not true or does not apply, just say "Does not apply."

Step 3:
When client is settled and ready, then place your hand, palm toward the client 6 to 12 inches out from the pubic area.
State "Visualize red - a stop sign red, ruby red." Wait a moment. Say "OK?" and let the patient acknowledge visualizing the color.
Directing your attention to the client make the statement: "Some days, life is just not worth living." Wait for a response.

"Some days I feel like throwing in the towel."
Wait for a response.
"I do not feel safe."
Wait for a response.
"My needs are not met".
Wait for a response.

<u>Step 4</u>:
Now move the palm up towards the sacral chakra.
Tell your client to visualize terra cotta orange / brown.
Wait for client to confirm that she / he is visualizing the color.
Say "I do not feel sexy."
Wait for a response.
"The best things in life always go to someone else."
Wait for a response.
"My life is not recognized or appreciated."
Wait for a response.

<u>Step 5</u>:
Now raise your hand, palm still facing the client, up to the solar plexus.
Have your client visualize a bright, sunshine yellow.
Make the following statements.
"Everyone walks all over me."
Wait for a response.
"I'm not living the job or thing that I love."
Wait for a response.
"I have no power in my life."

Wait for a response.

<u>Step 6</u>:
Now move the palm up to the heart area.
Have the client visualize a deep green.
Make the statement.
"I am not loved."
Wait for a response.
"I forget what it feels like to feel love."
Wait for a response.
"I cannot give or receive love."
Wait for a response.

Now tell the client he or she is going to be asked to acknowledge his or her inner beings. If the client does not recognize any one of them, he or she should simply respond that the statement does not apply.

"Now bring forth your inner child."

**

"What do you see?" You may need to prompt with questions such as "How is she dressed? Is she happy, etc.?"
Wait for a response.
"Does she have anything to say to you?"
Wait for a response.
"Anything else?"
Wait for a response.
"OK, let her fly away to the green room."

**

Repeat the questions between the "**" three more times, for the inner teen, woman, and man.

Now bring forth your inner teen. (from ** to **)
Now bring forth your inner woman. (from ** to **)
Now bring forth your inner man. (from ** to **)

Step 7:
Now move your palm up to the throat chakra.
Have your client visualize blue.
Make the following statements.
"No one listens to a word I say."
Wait for a response.
"My arts and crafts are second-rate."
Wait for a response.
"Nobody values my ideas and insights."
Wait for a response.

Step 8:
Now move your palm up to the third eye.
Have your client visualize purple.
Make the following statements.
"I am not intuitive."
Wait for a response.
"I am not able to access my inner wisdom."
Wait for a response.

<u>Step 9</u>:
Now move your palm up to the crown chakra.
Have your client visualize white.
"I'm not connected with Divine Source."
Wait for a response.
"I am separated from God."
Wait for a response.

<u>Step 10</u>:
Now bring the palm down to the base chakra.
Have the client visualize red.
Make the following statements and say "Repeat the following statements exactly as I say them."
"I embrace life and live it abundantly."
Wait for a response.
"I am safe."
Wait for a response.
"My needs are met."
Wait for a response.

<u>Step 11</u>:
Move the palm up to sacral chakra.
Have the client visualize terra cotta.
Make the following statements.
"I am sexy."
Wait for a response. (You may need to coach the client to repeat the statement.)
"The best things in life always come my way."
Wait for a response.
"My wants and needs are met."
Wait for a response.

<u>Step 12</u>:
Move the palm up to the solar plexus.
Have the client visualize yellow.
Make the following statements.
"I set boundaries and others respect them."
Wait for a response.
"I have valuable ideas."
Wait for a response.
"I have authority and mastery of my life."
Wait for a response.

<u>Step 13</u>:
Move your palm up to the heart chakra.
Have your client visualize green.
Have your client repeat out loud.
"I am fully loved."
Wait for a response.
"I love fully."
Wait for a response.

(Note to practitioner: At this point you are going to ask the client to call forth again his or her inner child, teen, woman, and man. Call forth all four individually, even if the client stated, in the initial step, that any of them did not apply.)

"Now bring forth your inner child from the green room."

**

"What do you see?"
Wait for a response.
"Is there anything she wants to say to you?"
Wait for a response.
"Anything else?"
Wait for a response.
"Let her fly away to where ever she wants to go."
**

Repeat the questions between the "**" three more times, for the inner teen, woman, and man.

Now bring forth your inner teen. (from ** to **)
Now bring forth your inner woman. (from ** to **)
Now bring forth your inner man. (from ** to **)

Step 14:
Now move your hand up to the throat chakra.
Have your client visualize a pure blue like the skies or the oceans.
Have them say out loud.
"I speak my truth."
Wait for a response.

<u>Step 15</u>:
Now move the palm up to the third eye.
Have the client visualize indigo.
Have client repeat out loud.
"I see."
Wait for a response.
"I now access the power of my intuitive mind."
Wait for a response.
"I have clear insight."
Wait for a response.

<u>Step 16</u>:
Now move the palm up to the crown.
Have the client visualize violet white and repeat out loud.
"I now access my spiritual wisdom, my connection to the divine."

<u>Step 17</u>:
Withdraw hands from client's field. Wait a moment and ask the client how he or she feels. If this was done correctly, the response will be "light" or "refreshed."

CHAPTER SEVEN
Grounding, GAPS, Cord Cutting

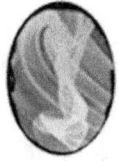

There are any number of ways for the healer to cleanse, attune or protect him or herself. Simple methods are desired and better than complicated and complex ones. The three suggested here are: Grounding, Gaps, and Cord Cutting (severing ties). After doing them a few times you will be able to do them quickly, almost automatically in your mind.

Grounding

Grounding yourself is done to connect you to your root chakra. This is important as the root chakra is also known as the liver of the chakra system. It is associated with the color black. It is responsible for the detoxification of energetic toxins.

This is best done with bare feet on the ground or at the very least with shoes off, remembering the properties of leather from the earlier chapters.

1) Close eyes and attain a comfortable stance with feet apart on the floor

2) Sense the feet sinking down into the ground

3) Now imagine from the soles of your feet, golden roots growing down into the earth.

4) They grow deep and gnarly, strong and wide.

5) The deeper they get, the stronger they get, so that no matter the force of the wind above, you stand firm.

6) When you feel totally anchored and secure, open your eyes slowly and take a deep breath.

You are now grounded.

GAPS

GAPS is a second self-healing/rejuevenating technique that all healers should perform on themselves once a day, if not more frequently.

Ground
Attune / Ask
Protect
Say thanks

Ground: (as above)

Ask: Ask your angels, guides, totems or heavenly helpers – whoever you work with to attend and assist
Attune: Align yourself with your higher power.

If you believe God is without, imagine that on the top of your head, just above the crown chakra, there is a white translucent cloud, the purest white you have ever seen. Now draw the cloud down through your crown chakra, and let it fill your whole body like a liquid syrup, filling every crevice, until you are filled to overflowing.

Or, if you believe that God is within, sense your heart chakra. See it glow. Allow the Light to flow out from the heart chakra to every cell of your being until you are totally filled with pure Light.

<u>Protect</u>: Surround yourself with a glowy, translucent egg. It is your protective capsule. When you step sideways, it moves with you; when you sit, it sits with you. Nothing can enter your egg and you are completely surrounded and continually infused with the power within it. Now, if you wish, sprinkle the outside of the egg with diamond dust, a protective coat.

<u>Say Thanks</u>: Thank your Higher Power and your spiritual helpers.

Cord Cutting

This is also sometimes called "severing ties."

As we go through life, we all make energetic cords / attachments to people, events, and things. We've all heard the expressions:

He's tied to his mother's apron strings.
She pulls at the strings of my heart.
She's got him on a short leash.
No strings attached.
She's stringing him along.

You may think these are just figures of speech, but think again.

Whenever you interact with a person, place or thing, you create an energetic cord with that person, place or thing. Over time, these cords whither off with disuse, or can flourish and grow with continued exposure or by remembering it.

While some cords serve a purpose, most do not. Most cause dependency or energy drainage. As long as you are connected by a person, place or thing, you can at any time be drawn into its energy and find yourself inexplicably drained, sad, mad, etc. Energy healers especially have to be careful not to become drained themselves. Most energy healers cut cords on a regular basis. It is easy to do. You just have to remember to do it.

Be in a quiet, safe place where you know you'll be undisturbed.

Close your eyes and sense your torso.

Slowly scan it with your mind's eye – do you sense any spot that should not be there? Do you sense a spot that is hot, or cold, or heavy, or staticy or dull? Is anything amiss?

Now zero in on that spot and isolate it.

Next you need to separate your body from the spot. In your mind's eye cut the spot out, lift it out, or burn it out - whatever removal method works best for you.

Watch it fall from your body, dissolving into butterflies that flutter away.
Repeat this on any other spot that you find. You should do cord cutting on a regular basis.

As you begin to do it a little more often, you will begin to notice a face, a time, a place associated with these cords. . You may have a quick video or audio flash. Perhaps a scent might jog your memory. Some people just have a knowing. Some have a combination.

Conclusion

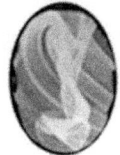

So as you see, you CAN do it. You can be the confident, professional you want to be.

You are responsible for keeping yourself rested and well so that the healing life force energy that flows through is pure and of optimal quality.

You are responsible for "setting the stage"/creating the ambiance.

Now take a deep breath in and a deep breath out. Let go and let Spirit flow through you.

Don't be surprised if you see an angel-or two along the way.